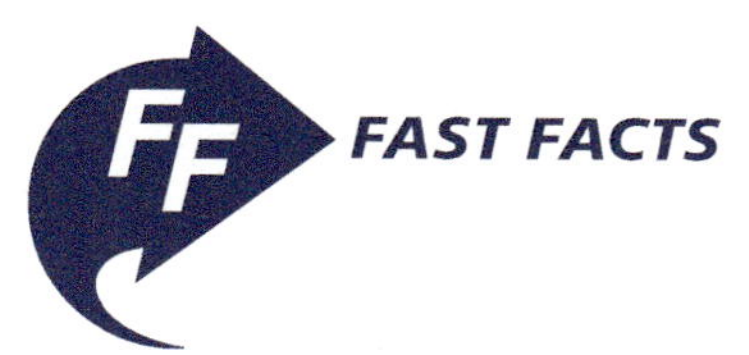

# Measurable Residual Disease

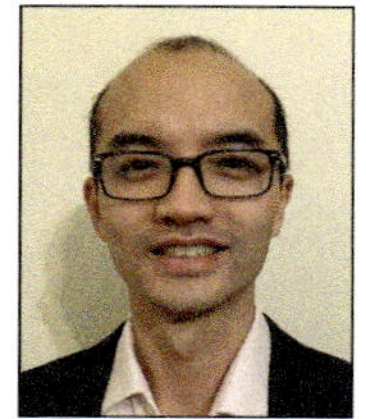

**Justin Loke** BM BCh PhD MRCP FRCPath
Clinical Trials Fellow
CRUK Clinical Trials Unit, Birmingham and
Queen Elizabeth Hospital, Birmingham, UK

**Declaration of Independence**
This book is as balanced and as practical as we can make it.
Ideas for improvement are always welcome: fastfacts@karger.com

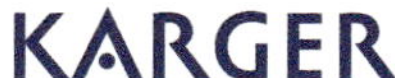

Fast Facts: Measurable Residual Disease
First published 2020



S. Karger Publishers Ltd, Elizabeth House, Queen Street, Abingdon,
Oxford OX14 3LN, UK
Tel: +44 (0)1235 523233

Book orders can be placed by telephone or email, or via the website.
Please telephone +41 61 306 1440 or email orders@karger.com
To order via the website, please go to karger.com



A CIP record for this title is available from the British Library.

ISBN: 978-3-318-06824-5

Loke J (Justin)
Fast Facts: Measurable Residual Disease/
Justin Loke

Medical illustrations by Graeme Chambers, Belfast, UK.
Typesetting by S. Karger Publishers Ltd, Abingdon, UK.
Printed in the UK with Xpedient Print.

# List of abbreviations

**ALL:** acute lymphoblastic leukemia

**AML:** acute myeloid leukemia

**APML:** acute promyelocytic leukemia

**CBF:** core binding factor (AML)

**CHIP:** clonal hematopoiesis of indeterminate potential

**CLL:** chronic lymphocytic leukemia

**CML:** chronic myeloid leukemia

**CR:** complete remission

**CR1:** first complete response

**DNA:** deoxyribonucleic acid

**ELN:** European LeukemiaNet

**FDA:** (US) Food and Drug Administration

**FISH:** fluorescent in situ hybridization

**MRD:** measurable residual disease (also referred to as minimal residual disease)

**NGS:** next-generation DNA sequencing

**NICE:** (England and Wales) National Institute for Health and Care Excellence

**OS:** overall survival

**PFS:** progression-free survival

**Ph+/–:** Philadelphia chromosome positive/negative

**RT-qPCR:** quantitative reverse transcriptase polymerase chain reaction

# Introduction

Conventional methods of detecting disease remission in cancers such as leukemia rely on microscopic analysis of tissue samples. Measurable (or minimal) residual disease (MRD) describes the presence of disease beyond the levels of sensitivity afforded by microscopy.

*Fast Facts: Measurable Residual Disease* describes what is meant by MRD, the opportunities and challenges afforded by its identification and the advantages and disadvantages of the methods used for its detection. Specific examples are given to illustrate the implications of detecting MRD in different disease scenarios, with emphasis on acute myeloid and lymphoblastic leukemias.

With the recognition and monitoring of MRD likely to play an increasingly important role in disease prognosis and subsequent treatment direction, this accessible resource is ideal for any healthcare professional wanting to know more about this exciting and fast-moving area.

# 1 What is measurable residual disease?

As every patient has a different response to treatment, a fundamental question is how to assess this treatment response. The assessment of response to treatment has enormous implications for what the patient can expect for the future and whether they might require further monitoring or treatment. For some malignancies such as lymphoma, imaging to assess tumor size will be critical. However, for leukemias, which are fundamentally diseases of the blood and bone marrow, there can be many levels of assessment.

The simplest level is that of the full blood count – has the count been corrected so that the patient can become independent of blood and platelet transfusion support?

The next level is that of the bone marrow. Assessment can take place using light microscopy so that the hematologist/pathologist can physically count cells to determine whether there is complete remission (CR; sometimes referred to as morphological remission). In acute myeloid leukemia (AML), for example, CR is said to have occurred if blasts account for fewer than 5% of cells overall.[1] Below the level of sensitivity afforded by this direct physical assessment, it is difficult to ascertain by microscopy alone whether any leukemic cells remain. Despite cells having the characteristic appearance of a 'blast', it is not always clear whether they are normal regenerating stem/progenitor cells or residual leukemic disease. The implications are clear in acute leukemia: patients often achieve CR, as assessed by light microscopy, after initial induction chemotherapy, but they inevitably relapse in the absence of further treatment.

Critically, the assessment of measurable (historically called minimal) residual disease (MRD) allows a dynamic evaluation of a patient's risk of relapse and treatment failure over time, beyond the initial assessment of risk based on genetic and clinical factors. It is to be hoped that this will inform patient/clinician discussions about disease management options.

## Assessing measurable residual disease

Assessments developed to quantify MRD are based on a range of sensitive techniques that, essentially, detect small numbers of disease cells. Improved sensitivity allows better prognostication and treatment stratification for patients. The move from describing this residual disease as 'minimal' to 'measurable' is predicated on the findings of studies that have shown 'minimal' to be misleading, as its presence tends to be associated with poor prognosis.

MRD assessment, like all tests, is subject to limitations: a negative MRD result does not necessarily mean a patient is cured, nor does a positive MRD result imply relapse will definitely occur. The different levels of disease quantification and the limits of different forms of assessment are shown in Figure 1.1.

MRD technology is based on the identification of a disease marker (for example, a surface protein or DNA mutation) at diagnosis that can be quantified during treatment. Ideally, this marker should remain stably present on or in the cell throughout the disease course.

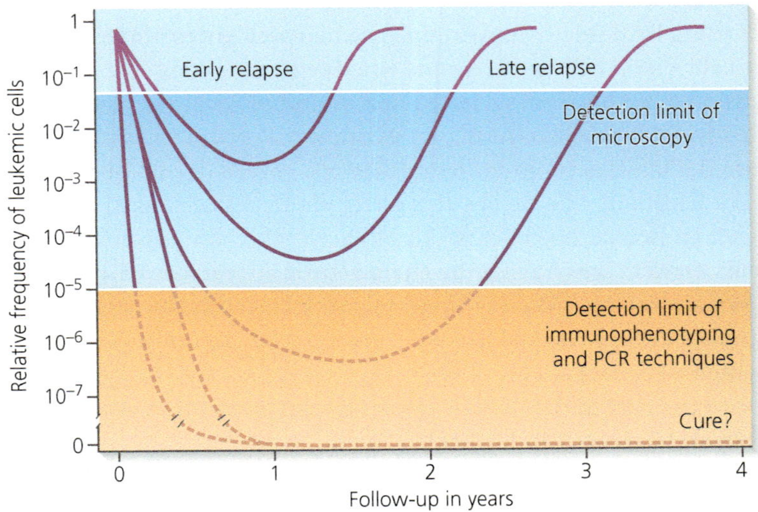


**Figure 1.1** The clinical trajectories and associated levels of measurable residual disease that are possible for a patient with acute lymphoblastic leukemia. PCR, polymerase chain reaction. Adapted from van Dongen et al. 2015.[2]

MRD techniques are developing rapidly, but a brief overview of the different methods is given in the next chapter.

**CR with MRD negativity** has been suggested as a new form of CR in many clinical trial response criteria.[1] It may also be increasingly useful in conditions such as chronic lymphocytic leukemia (CLL), where the treatments are now extremely effective and it is difficult to show significant differences in overall survival in clinical trials. This is also referred to as a 'surrogate endpoint'.

**Challenges.** Each test needs to be calibrated to a certain standard and performed in a reproducible manner to ensure the level of sensitivity. Interpreting the results depends on expertise. As a consequence, MRD samples may need to go to regional or national laboratories for analysis. There is also the expense of collecting, processing and interpreting the information.

National trial protocols, particularly those developed for acute lymphoblastic leukemia (ALL) and AML, have helped clinicians act on results of MRD analysis. International collaborations such as European LeukemiaNet (ELN) have produced helpful guidelines. Chronic myeloid leukemia (CML) is characterized by the presence of a t(9;22) chromosomal translocation which produces a fusion protein BCR–ABL1. The fusion transcripts from the fusion gene *BCR–ABL1* can be used to monitor the presence of disease. ELN guidelines have been produced to support the interpretation of *BCR–ABL1* results.[3] Similarly, international collaborations have attempted to set best-practice standards for MRD assessment in AML.[4]

**Limitations.** Many MRD technologies are specific for disease subtypes. MRD assessment is not suitable for all disease subtypes, and alternative forms of disease assessment are required (for example, imaging and histology). Also, MRD may be prognostic, but it is not always clear how this should influence therapy. For example, it is not known whether intensifying treatment for patients with MRD before an allogeneic stem cell transplant necessarily improves outcomes. Finally, MRD quantification (the degree of MRD) needs to be interpreted within the context of the type of specimen, disease, mutation and treatment and patient factors.

**Patient considerations.** Awaiting the results of MRD assessment can be an anxious time for the patient, who also has the stress and inconvenience of repeat blood or bone marrow sampling. MRD positivity and negativity need to be communicated clearly. A negative MRD result does not necessarily mean the patient is cured, though it may increase the chance of achieving a cure over time. Similarly, a positive MRD result does not necessarily mean that they have relapsed, but the risk of relapse may be increased.

**Key points – what is measurable residual disease?**

- Measurable (or minimal) residual disease (MRD) refers to the low number of disease cells that may remain despite the patient being in remission.
- Different methods of MRD assessment have distinct advantages and disadvantages.
- Results need to be interpreted based on many factors, including the testing method as well as the patient and disease context. Guidelines are available to help interpret MRD levels.

**References**

1. Döhner H, Estey E, Grimwade D et al. Diagnosis and management of AML in adults: 2017 ELN recommendations from an international expert panel. *Blood* 2017;129:424–47.

2. van Dongen JJ, van der Velden VH, Brüggeman M, Orfao A. Minimal residual disease diagnostics in acute lymphoblastic leukemia: need for sensitive, fast, and standardized technologies. *Blood* 2015;125: 3996–4009.

3. Baccarani M, Deininger MW, Rosti G et al. European LeukemiaNet recommendations for the management of chronic myeloid leukemia: 2013. *Blood* 2013;122: 872–84.

4. Schuurhuis GJ, Heuser M, Freeman S et al. Minimal/measurable residual disease in AML: a consensus document from the European LeukemiaNet MRD Working Party. *Blood* 2018;131:1275–91.

# 2 How is MRD measured?

There is no single optimal measurement of measurable residual disease (MRD). In this chapter, we describe the principles behind some of the common and emerging techniques and discuss the advantages and disadvantages of each one. One common point is that dilution of the bone marrow with blood (hemodilution) can affect the results (just as a diluted sample might affect the morphological assessment). Therefore, a common recommendation is that the 'first pull' bone marrow is used for MRD analysis.

The advantages and disadvantages of different methods of MRD measurement are summarized in Figure 2.1.

## Multiparameter flow cytometry

Flow cytometry is a technique whereby antibodies are used to bind to different cell markers on the outside (and sometimes on the inside) of cells. Individual antibodies bind specifically to target proteins. These antibodies are tagged (conjugated) with a fluorescent molecule called a fluorochrome. The treated cells then pass, cell by cell, through a laser beam. If the cell is coated with the antibody, the fluorochrome emits a specific signal that is detected by the flow cytometer. This allows the identification of specific proteins present on the cell. To identify different populations of cells (such as leukemic cells and T cells), multiple fluorochrome-conjugated antibodies that can bind to different targets are used. These groups of antibodies may be described as a panel.

Panels of fluorochrome-conjugated antibodies are designed for different diseases (for example, the antibody panel designed for acute myeloid leukemia [AML] is different from that designed for chronic lymphocytic leukemia [CLL]). These panels typically include eight different targets, though some laboratories use multiple panels and can detect more targets.

Different analytic techniques are possible: for example, one way of analyzing AML cells is to look for specific abnormal expression

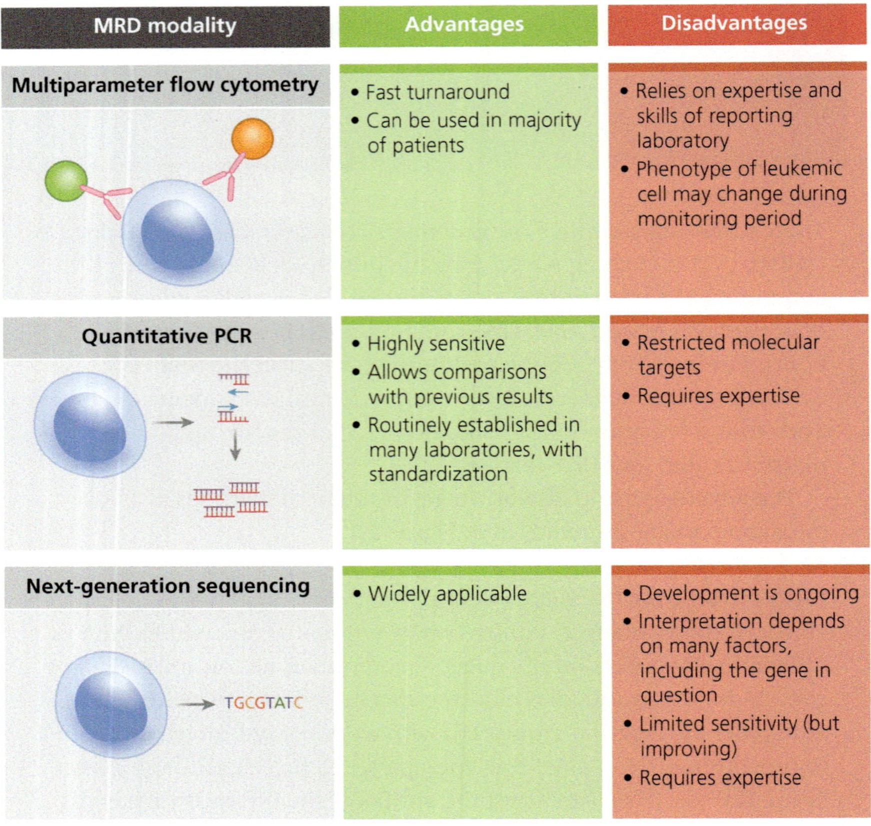

| MRD modality | Advantages | Disadvantages |
|---|---|---|
| Multiparameter flow cytometry | • Fast turnaround<br>• Can be used in majority of patients | • Relies on expertise and skills of reporting laboratory<br>• Phenotype of leukemic cell may change during monitoring period |
| Quantitative PCR | • Highly sensitive<br>• Allows comparisons with previous results<br>• Routinely established in many laboratories, with standardization | • Restricted molecular targets<br>• Requires expertise |
| Next-generation sequencing | • Widely applicable | • Development is ongoing<br>• Interpretation depends on many factors, including the gene in question<br>• Limited sensitivity (but improving)<br>• Requires expertise |



**Figure 2.1** The advantages and disadvantages of the main methods used to analyze measurable residual disease (MRD). AML, acute myeloid leukemia; PCR, polymerase chain reaction.

patterns of surface markers at diagnosis and then track these markers, and hence the cells, through treatment. In some patients, though, some cell markers may be lost and so this technique may miss changes in the appearance or profile (phenotype) of the cells during treatment. A combination of techniques to enable capture of both diagnostic and relapse-associated phenotypes is recommended.

**Advantages.** The benefit of this technique is that it can capture other information, such as the viability of the cell sample – whether cells are alive, rapidly proliferating or dead. Also, because a range of markers are analyzed, the results can provide a perspective on the identity of the cell. For example, one area of interest in AML is the identification of leukemic stem cell populations. Leukemic stem cells are thought to be a reservoir of cells that may be resistant to chemotherapy; persistence of these cells can lead to relapse, with blasts forming the bulk of the leukemia.[1,2] Many ways have been used to describe leukemic stem cells, including the presence on their cell surface of different protein markers. It is unsurprising that researchers have tried to correlate the presence of different leukemic cells with outcomes. Using flow cytometry to monitor the leukemic stem cell population and to assess MRD has been shown to have additional prognostic value for some patients before allogeneic stem cell transplant.[3]

The fast turnaround of the sample is also an advantage of this technique. Most laboratories can run the test within 24 hours of receiving the sample, though interpretation of the results may take longer.

**Limitations.** Although flow cytometry is a readily available technique in many laboratories, selecting the correct panel of antibodies and the subsequent analysis and interpretation of the results depend on expertise. Consequently, not all laboratories can perform multiparameter flow cytometry for MRD assessment.

### Polymerase chain reaction

Quantitative reverse transcriptase polymerase chain reaction (RT-qPCR) is a standard molecular biological technique. DNA is amplified and the copies of the target sequence are detected using a fluorescent marker that binds newly synthesized DNA strands in the reaction, allowing quantification (Figure 2.2).

As a starting point, a target needs to be identified. This is usually a known mutated gene. The polymerase enzyme copies this target using a set of primers, synthesized to match the start and end of the target sequence, and free nucleotides. Repeated cycles are performed to produce multiple copies of the target. To quantify the DNA, the number of copies produced is compared with the levels of a standard, often a housekeeper gene (one that is essential for cell function and is therefore expressed at a reproducibly constant level). The starting

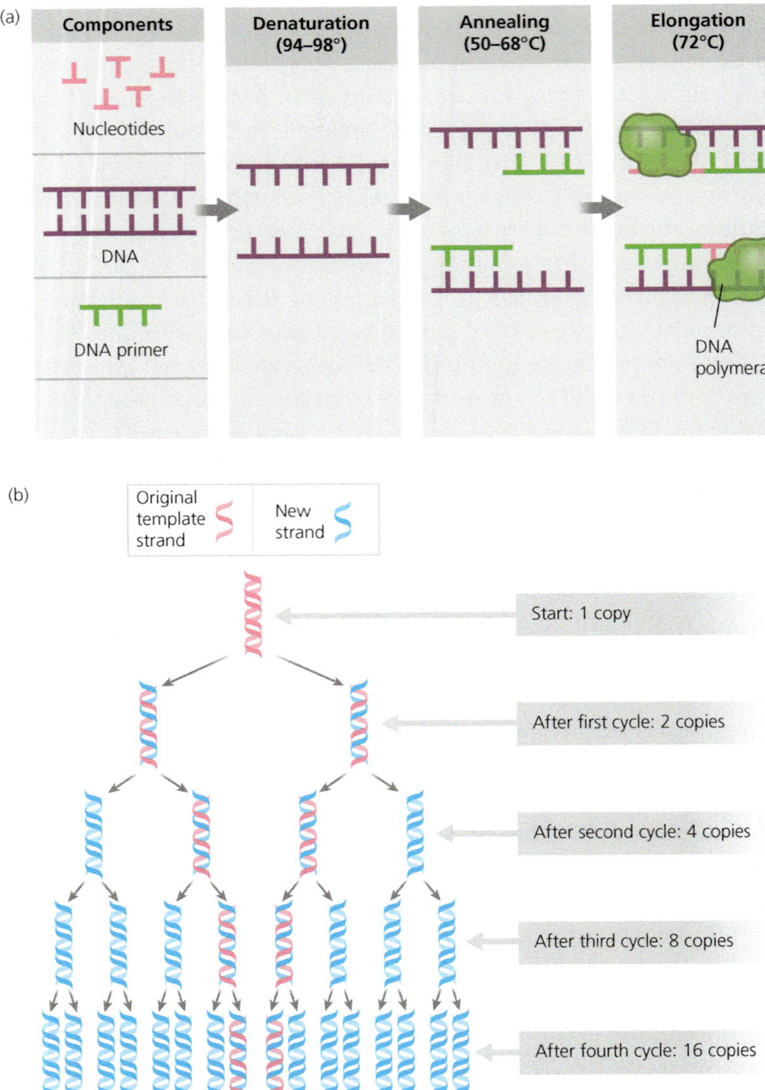


**Figure 2.2** (a) Using primers that are complementary to the target sequence allows the polymerase enzyme to produce a new strand of complementary DNA. (b) The polymerase chain reaction results in an exponential increase in the number of DNA strands, which can be quantified against a standard.

quantity of mutant DNA is calculated in comparison with the standard, and a level of disease can be inferred.

**Applications.** RT-qPCR is firmly established in clinical practice for certain diseases: for example, in the monitoring of the *PML–RARA* fusion transcripts in acute promyelocytic leukemia (APML) and *BCR–ABL1* fusion transcripts in chronic myeloid leukemia (CML) and acute lymphoblastic leukemia (ALL) (fusion transcripts arise when a mutation brings together two unrelated genes to produce a new fusion gene). These applications are well standardized with good quality control methods implemented, so results are consistent across international centers. With many monitoring targets, the sensitivity is greater than with flow cytometry and the target can be quantified to very low levels such as 1 in 100 000 cells.

RT-qPCR is also used to track the disease course in ALL. Indeed, this type of RT-qPCR is the primary form of MRD assessment in ALL and is more widely used than multiparameter flow cytometry. Normally, each lymphocyte expresses a particular T-cell receptor/immunoglobulin that allows it to bind specifically to a target. This specificity arises as a consequence of the immune system evolving to recognize a panoply of foreign pathogens. During lymphocyte development, the genetic material used as a general template for the receptor/immunoglobulin is cut and edited differently to produce a specific receptor/immunoglobulin. This unique identifier can be used to identify a cell as being clonal (a clonal population comprises identical cells arising from a single cell precursor), as happens in leukemic populations. RT-qPCR can be used to monitor the specific genetic rearrangements associated with particular receptors/immunoglobulins, and the technique gives sensitive detection of disease levels during the course of treatment.

When leukemia progresses, further secondary mutations can lead to the development of different subpopulations – subclones – of cancerous cells. As subclones may be lost during treatment because of selection pressures, it is good practice, where possible, to monitor more than one receptor/immunoglobulin genetic rearrangement.

**Limitations.** Determining the specific genetic rearrangements requires expertise. It is important that the correct diagnostic samples reach the

MRD laboratory so that the rearrangements can be identified (many diseases specifically require bone marrow). This is important as, without the correct sample from before treatment, an MRD laboratory may subsequently be unable to identify a marker for MRD monitoring.

The results of RT-qPCR often take days to weeks to come through, as the experiments are often performed in batches. The results then have to be validated and authorized by the clinical scientist. Interpretation also often requires knowledge of the preceding result, among many other factors, and sequential testing may be needed to ensure detection of disease that progresses on a molecular level.

In AML, there is not a clear target for RT-qPCR in all disease subtypes. Targets that are well characterized include:

- *PML–RARA*
- mutations affecting *NPM1*, encoding nucleophosmin (NPM1), that give rise to the mutated protein NPM1-cytoplasmic (NPM1c)
- *AML1–ETO* (also known as *RUNX1–RUNX1T1*)
- mutations giving rise to the fusion oncoprotein core binding factor β (CBFβ)–smooth muscle myosin heavy chain 11 (SMMHC)
- *MLL* fusion genes.

However, these mutations are present in only a minority of people with AML. That an RT-qPCR target is not present in the majority of people with AML limits the application of this technology.

## Next-generation DNA sequencing

**At diagnosis.** Next-generation DNA sequencing (NGS) is a new but well-established technology used at diagnosis. The technique is carried out in many clinical laboratories as a standard diagnostic procedure to identify mutations in either a few genes (targeted sequencing) or the entire genome. The ability to identify the genes that have prognostic value is particularly useful where the genetic heterogeneity of the disease is striking, such as in AML, and NGS is now firmly established in diagnosis and in prognostic algorithms. An AML with an *NPM1* mutation is, for example, likely to have a very different response to treatment from that of an AML with a mutation in the *RUNX1* gene.

Although NGS requires a number of different experimental steps, it is now performed routinely. The DNA is initially broken down into smaller fragments; known sequences of DNA called adaptors (supplied by the manufacturer) are adjoined to the DNA fragments. This allows the small amount of DNA to be amplified using a polymerase enzyme similar to that used in RT-qPCR (see pages 15–18). The fragments of DNA with the adaptors can then attach to the surface of the sequencing machine. Millions of these fragments are read in parallel (at the same time) and the sequence of the DNA is reconstructed by bio-informaticians.

The cost of testing is falling rapidly. Often, samples from a number of patients are pooled into a single experimental run to minimize costs.

**To monitor MRD.** NGS may become a useful tool as it increases the number of patients with an MRD target that can be monitored, as nearly all patients will have an identifiable cancer-causing mutation. However, the utility of NGS as a technique to monitor MRD after a treatment course is not well established. Standardization of the technique for monitoring purposes, which is important for quality management, is still being developed.

Improvements to sensitivity are in development; currently, NGS is far behind RT-qPCR in its ability to detect very low levels of disease. The major limitation to sensitivity arises from an in-built sequencing error – the polymerase enzyme that is used has an error rate. Potentially, correcting for this error can increase sensitivity and hence the value of this assay in MRD monitoring.[4]

Furthermore, clinical interpretation of the results is still not clearly defined. For example, the detection of mutations in certain genes, such as *DNMT3A*, may not significantly affect prognosis because these mutations are also common in healthy elderly individuals. Clonal hematopoiesis of indeterminate potential (CHIP) is common with aging – genetically distinct subpopulations of cells with somatic mutations occur in the absence of hematologic disease.[5] The exclusion of these CHIP mutations is thought to improve the sensitivity of NGS MRD mutation analysis in AML MRD monitoring,[6] but such improvements have not been replicated consistently across studies.

## Other techniques

**Fluorescent in situ hybridization** (FISH) is another surrogate measurement of disease presence. This technique uses fluorescence-labeled 'probes', which are large stretches of DNA complementary to the target of interest. FISH is less sensitive than flow cytometry or RT-qPCR, but it can be useful for large chromosomal rearrangements and is more sensitive than routine chromosomal karyotyping. There is, however, a cost associated with the use of the probes and FISH also requires the time and skill of a clinical scientist to set up and interpret the tests.

**Chimerism.** Following transplantation, patients will have chimerism of their bone marrow or peripheral blood monitored. This is usually done by looking at polymorphisms in the donor cells and comparing them with those in the recipient cells. An example is PCR detection of recognized microsatellite regions, which are usually identified before the transplant and then used to track the donor:recipient cell mix in the transplanted hematopoietic system. This is not an MRD measurement, as it is not a disease marker in itself, but rapidly falling donor chimerism is associated with an increased risk of disease relapse.

## Sample requirements

Samples of bone marrow are often stipulated for MRD analysis, rather than blood (for example, in ALL monitoring). Many protocols for MRD assessment (for example, in AML and ALL) suggest using the first pull of bone marrow, with a set volume, to prevent sample hemodilution with peripheral blood, as this may affect the sensitivity of the measurement. For some tests, such as *BCR–ABL1* monitoring of CML in the chronic phase, monitoring of MRD using peripheral blood is acceptable.

## Key points – how is MRD measured?

- The optimal technique to assess measurable residual disease (MRD) depends on the patient and disease context, as each method has advantages and disadvantages.
- MRD measurement requires specialist laboratories but it is now widely standardized internationally.
- The most commonly used technologies are based on flow cytometry and quantitative reverse transcriptase polymerase chain reaction (RT-qPCR).
- Emerging technologies will likely provide new methods of disease assessment.

## References

1. Lapidot T, Sirard C, Vormoor J et al. A cell initiating human acute myeloid leukaemia after transplantation into SCID mice. *Nature* 1994;367:645–8.

2. Shlush LI, Mitchell A, Heisler L et al. Tracing the origins of relapse in acute myeloid leukaemia to stem cells. *Nature* 2017;547:104–8.

3. Bradbury C, Houlton AE, Akiki S et al. Prognostic value of monitoring a candidate immunophenotypic leukaemic stem/progenitor cell population in patients allografted for acute myeloid leukaemia. *Leukemia* 2015;29:988–91.

4. Thol F, Gabdoulline R, Liebich A et al. Measurable residual disease monitoring by NGS before allogeneic hematopoietic cell transplantation in AML. *Blood* 2018;132:1703–13.

5. Jaiswal S, Fontanillas P, Flannick J et al. Age-related clonal hematopoiesis associated with adverse outcomes. *N Engl J Med* 2014;371:2488–98.

6. Jongen-Lavrencic M, Grob T, Hanekamp D et al. Molecular minimal residual disease in acute myeloid leukemia. *N Engl J Med* 2018;378:1189–99.

# 3 What is the significance of MRD?

A result from testing for measurable residual disease (MRD) can be informative in different ways. At the simplest level, MRD testing can be used to determine prognosis. Most initial studies of MRD relied on showing that the presence of MRD correlated with increased relapse rates and reduced overall survival (OS). MRD can also be used to monitor therapy, but this depends on the availability of alternative therapeutic options. Finally, in some patients, MRD can be used to define an undetectable level of disease at which therapy may safely be de-escalated or stopped. This chapter focuses on the acute leukemias, for which the principles for MRD are best established. However, MRD monitoring is rapidly developing in chronic lymphocytic leukemia (CLL) and myeloma, and clinical trials will use MRD analysis with increasing frequency.

## Acute lymphoblastic leukemia

MRD monitoring in acute lymphoblastic leukemia (ALL), particularly in pediatric management, has been a paradigm for the use of this technology during treatment (Figure 3.1).

**In children**, outcomes have improved over recent decades, such that patients designated as low risk can have OS above 90%. MRD results have been used to determine the need for treatment de-escalation in patients with low-risk disease and treatment escalation for those with high-risk disease. This is founded on the establishment of MRD as a strong independent prognostic factor during treatment – for example, after induction chemotherapy – that can accurately inform the risk of disease relapse.

MRD assessment enables better personalization of treatment, thereby reducing treatment-related toxicities in patients for whom a less intensive management pathway is appropriate. The UKALL 2003 pediatric ALL treatment trial found that patients with low-risk ALL, as defined by a low/undetectable MRD at the end of induction therapy,

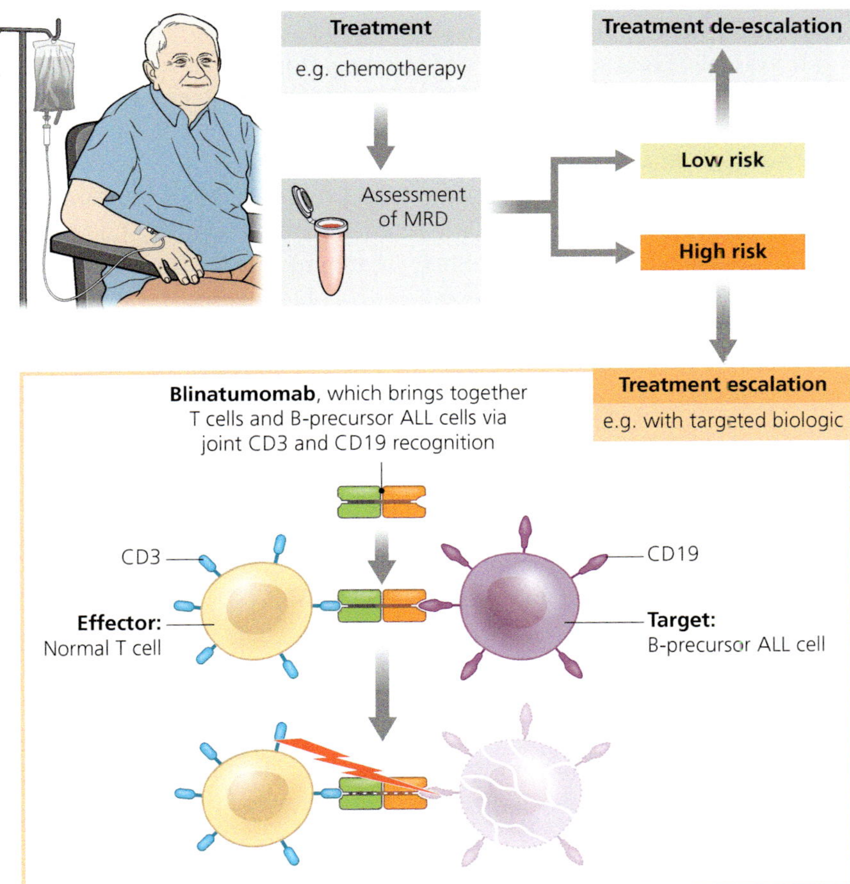


**Figure 3.1** Assessment of measurable residual disease after treatment is used to support decision-making for further treatment. ALL, acute lymphoblastic leukemia; MRD, measurable residual disease.

had equivalent outcomes whether they received one or two cycles of delayed intensification chemotherapy.[1] In contrast, patients with persistently high levels of MRD had better disease control with an augmented chemotherapy regimen.[2]

**In adults**, MRD is also a strong and independent prognostic factor in ALL. Some data suggest that patients with MRD do better with an allogeneic stem cell transplant than those unable to have a transplant (for example, because of the lack of a donor). However, data also suggest a poor outcome after transplant for patients who enter the treatment with MRD-positive disease.[3,4]

The first MRD-dependent treatment for ALL has been accepted by the National Institute for Health and Care Excellence (NICE [England and Wales]) and the Food and Drug Administration (FDA [USA]). Blinatumomab is a bispecific antibody that binds CD19, expressed on B-ALL cells, and CD3, expressed on T cells. Consequently, the antibody causes T cells to directly kill leukemic cells (see Figure 3.1). NICE recommends blinatumomab for patients with Philadelphia chromosome-negative (Ph–) B-ALL expressing CD19 in their first complete response (CR1) with an MRD level of at least 0.1%. This recommendation is based on a study showing that in patients in complete remission (CR) but with MRD, one cycle of blinatumomab treatment could produce high rates of response in terms of MRD (that is, MRD became undetectable).[5] Patients who had undetectable MRD after treatment with blinatumomab had improved OS.

Furthermore, MRD studies in ALL have shown the importance of interpreting the level of MRD based on the timepoint of measurement as well as the result itself. However, the difficulty of using MRD as a marker of disease is that its utility depends on an individual's preceding results and previous treatments and therefore results cannot be easily compared across different treatment protocols.

## Acute myeloid leukemia

The best-established use for MRD assessment in acute myeloid leukemia (AML) is in the management of acute promyelocytic leukemia (APML). This leukemia is characterized by the presence of the t(15;17) translocation that generates the *PML–RARA* fusion gene. The mutation can be detected by quantitative reverse transcriptase polymerase chain reaction (RT-qPCR) and its level used to monitor patients at the end of treatment; the presence of persistent or progressing MRD is a strong risk factor for relapse and an indication for salvage treatment.[6] As a result, the standard of care for these patients is to have 3-monthly bone marrow aspirates to check *PML–RARA* levels for 3 years. Salvage regimens include chemotherapy and arsenic trioxide.

**RT-qPCR monitoring** of *NPM1* mutations and chromosomal rearrangements inv(16) and t(8;21) (in core binding factor [CBF] AML) has also improved patient management, especially as these patients are often spared allogeneic stem cell transplantation as a result. Consequently, adequate monitoring is important for these individuals as they may have only limited cycles of chemotherapy.[7] There is a suggestion that performing 3-monthly bone marrow aspirates for 2 years is sufficient to detect impending relapse. This monitoring approach may, for example, allow the delivery of salvage therapy and stem cell transplant before overt relapse. If carried out after stem cell transplantation, monitoring can support the modification of immunosuppression and use of donor lymphocyte infusions.

Although mutant transcripts may still be present at remission in CBF AML, it is the degree of molecular response that is important: a 3-log reduction in MRD following the second course of chemotherapy is needed – without this there is a high risk of relapse. For some patients, MRD assessment may indicate that allogeneic stem cell transplantation is needed to consolidate the remission. However – illustrating the difficulties with applying these data – in a study testing the value of MRD, although relapse rates were far higher with increasing levels of MRD, the impact of the MRD result on survival was limited by the high rates of remission from salvage chemotherapy.[8] Running trials to test the use of MRD-directed treatment is challenging for many reasons, including participant numbers and suitable choices of intervention.

**Multiparameter flow cytometry** has also been shown to be a powerful prognostic marker in both younger and older patients with AML. In time, this may help improve the selection of those patients with intermediate-risk cytogenetic AML who should proceed to an allogeneic stem cell transplant. This is particularly important for patients who do not have a definitive prognostic cytogenetic or genetic mutation marker.[9] At present, MRD detected at or above 0.1% at timepoints after induction therapy, including pretransplantation, indicates a high risk of relapse. How this should direct treatment is a question tested in a number of clinical trials. The ongoing UK National Cancer Research Institute (NCRI) AML18 trial for elderly patients uses MRD assessment to direct treatment intensification.[10]

MRD has also been shown to be a strong prognostic marker before and after transplantation. The presence of MRD before an allogeneic stem cell transplant, detected using flow cytometry, has been shown to strongly affect outcomes.[11] Indeed, the data suggest that patients with MRD-positive disease who had an allogeneic stem cell transplant had poor outcomes similar to those of patients with morphologically detectable disease who underwent transplantation. Clearance of the mutation at an early timepoint after the transplant, detected by next-generation DNA sequencing (NGS), had implications for relapse risk.[12] However, at present, MRD assessment strategies need to be prospectively embedded in clinical trials to determine the optimal use of this technology. It is not yet clear, for example, whether improving patients' MRD response before the transplant – by intensifying conditioning regimens or giving pretransplant consolidation chemotherapy – will improve outcomes.

Finally, it may be that a combination of these MRD-monitoring technologies will be used in the future to optimally manage patients with AML. A large study of patients with AML has shown that flow cytometry and NGS monitoring of MRD have additive prognostic power.[13]

## Use of MRD in other diseases

Analysis of MRD is increasingly used in myeloma and CLL treatment. Novel methods are being developed. One example is the assessment of circulating tumor DNA from patients' plasma, a technique that has been developed largely in the solid tumor and lymphoma field. This is useful in CLL, where nodal disease is a burden. The effectiveness of new treatment combinations for CLL has necessitated a longer assessment period to ascertain progression-free survival (PFS) in comparisons of new treatment strategies. There have been developments by regulatory authorities to allow the use of CR with MRD negativity to 1 in 10 000 cells as a criterion they will consider while the full PFS is ascertained. It is hoped that this will allow effective drugs to be evaluated more rapidly.

In myeloma treatment, flow cytometry has been used to assess MRD for a considerable period of time. However, many patients have relapsed following a result of 'MRD-undetectable disease'. Advances in flow cytometry have led to improvements in MRD measurements and alternatives now exist, including NGS to identify and quantify immunoglobulin rearrangements. As in other areas of hematology, the need for MRD assessment has been driven by the need for a discriminating response criterion for the increasing number of therapies with high conventionally measured response rates. This will, in turn, lead to the assessment of MRD-directed therapy in upcoming clinical trials.

**Key points – what is the significance of MRD?**

- Risk stratification using measurable residual disease (MRD) is important for patients undergoing intensive treatment.
- MRD is a key decision driver in acute lymphoblastic leukemia (ALL), especially in pediatrics, to ensure the right intensity of treatment and for optimal timing of treatments.
- MRD monitoring is important for detecting and preventing relapse of overt disease in acute myeloid leukemia (AML), particularly in acute promyelocytic leukemia (APML).
- MRD monitoring is now a key part of risk stratification in most clinical trials involving patients with leukemia or myeloma.

**References**

1. Vora A, Goulden N, Wade R et al. Treatment reduction for children and young adults with low-risk acute lymphoblastic leukaemia defined by minimal residual disease (UKALL 2003): a randomised controlled trial. *Lancet Oncol* 2013;14:199–209.

2. Vora A, Goulden N, Mitchell C et al. Augmented post-remission therapy for a minimal residual disease-defined high-risk subgroup of children and young people with clinical standard-risk and intermediate-risk acute lymphoblastic leukaemia (UKALL 2003): a randomised controlled trial. *Lancet Oncol* 2014;15:809–18.

3. Ribera JM, Oriol A, Morgades M et al. Treatment of high-risk Philadelphia chromosome-negative acute lymphoblastic leukemia in adolescents and adults according to early cytologic response and minimal residual disease after consolidation assessed by flow cytometry: final results of the PETHEMA ALL-AR-03 trial. *J Clin Oncol* 2014;32:1595–604.

4. Logan AC, Vashi N, Faham M et al. Immunoglobulin and T cell receptor gene high-throughput sequencing quantifies minimal residual disease in acute lymphoblastic leukemia and predicts post-transplantation relapse and survival. *Biol Blood Marrow Transplant* 2014;20:1307–13.

5. Gökbuget N, Dombret H, Bonifacio M et al. Blinatumomab for minimal residual disease in adults with B-cell precursor acute lymphoblastic leukemia. *Blood* 2018;131:1522–31.

6. Grimwade D, Jovanovic JV, Hills RK et al. Prospective minimal residual disease monitoring to predict relapse of acute promyelocytic leukemia and to direct pre-emptive arsenic trioxide therapy. *J Clin Oncol* 2009;27:3650–8.

7. Ivey A, Hills RK, Simpson MA et al. Assessment of minimal residual disease in standard-risk AML. *N Engl J Med* 2016;374:422–33.

8. Jourdan E, Boissel N, Chevret S et al. Prospective evaluation of gene mutations and minimal residual disease in patients with core binding factor acute myeloid leukemia. *Blood* 2013;121:2213–23.

9. Freeman SD, Hills RK, Virgo P et al. Measurable residual disease at induction redefines partial response in acute myeloid leukemia and stratifies outcomes in patients at standard risk without *NPM1* mutations. *J Clin Oncol* 2018; 36:1486–97.

10. Freeman SD, Virgo P, Couzens S et al. Prognostic relevance of treatment response measured by flow cytometric residual disease detection in older patients with acute myeloid leukemia. *J Clin Oncol* 2013;31: 4123–31.

11. Araki D, Wood BL, Othus M et al. Allogeneic hematopoietic cell transplantation for acute myeloid leukemia: time to move toward a minimal residual disease-based definition of complete remission? *J Clin Oncol* 2016;34:329–36.

12. Kim T, Moon JH, Ahn JS et al. Next-generation sequencing-based posttransplant monitoring of acute myeloid leukemia identifies patients at high risk of relapse. *Blood* 2018;132:1604–13.

13. Jongen-Lavrencic M, Grob T, Hanekamp D et al. Molecular minimal residual disease in acute myeloid leukemia. *N Engl J Med* 2018;378:1189–99.

# Useful resources

### UK

**Blood Cancer UK**
www.bloodcancer.org.uk

**Cancer Research UK**
www.cancerresearchuk.org

**Children with Cancer UK**
www.childrenwithcancer.org.uk

**Leukaemia Cancer Society**
www.leukaemiacancersociety.org

**Leukaemia Care**
www.leukaemiacare.org.uk

**Leukaemia & Myeloma Research UK**
www.lmruk.org

**Leukaemia UK**
www.leukaemiauk.org.uk

**Myeloma UK**
Myeloma.org.uk

### USA

**American Cancer Society**
www.cancer.org

**Leukemia & Lymphoma Society**
www.lls.org

**Leukemia Research Foundation**
www.allbloodcancers.org

**Multiple Myeloma Research Foundation**
www.themmrf.org

**The Myeloma Beacon**
www.myelomabeacon.com

### International

**International Myeloma Foundation**
www.myeloma.org

**Leukaemia and Blood Cancer New Zealand**
www.leukaemia.org.nz

**Leukaemia Foundation (Australia)**
www.leukaemia.org.au

**Leukemia and Lymphoma Society Canada**
www.llscanada.org

**Myeloma Australia**
www.myeloma.org.au

**Myeloma Canada**
www.myelomacanada.ca

## *FastTest*

**You've read the book ... now test yourself with key questions from the authors**

- Go to the FastTest for this title ***FREE*** **at karger.com/fastfacts**
- Approximate time **10 minutes**
- For best retention of the key issues, try taking the FastTest before and after reading

# Index